Diabetic Air Fryer Delights

Easy and Healthy Recipes
for the Air Fryer
to Prevent and Control Diabetes

Lilith Ballard

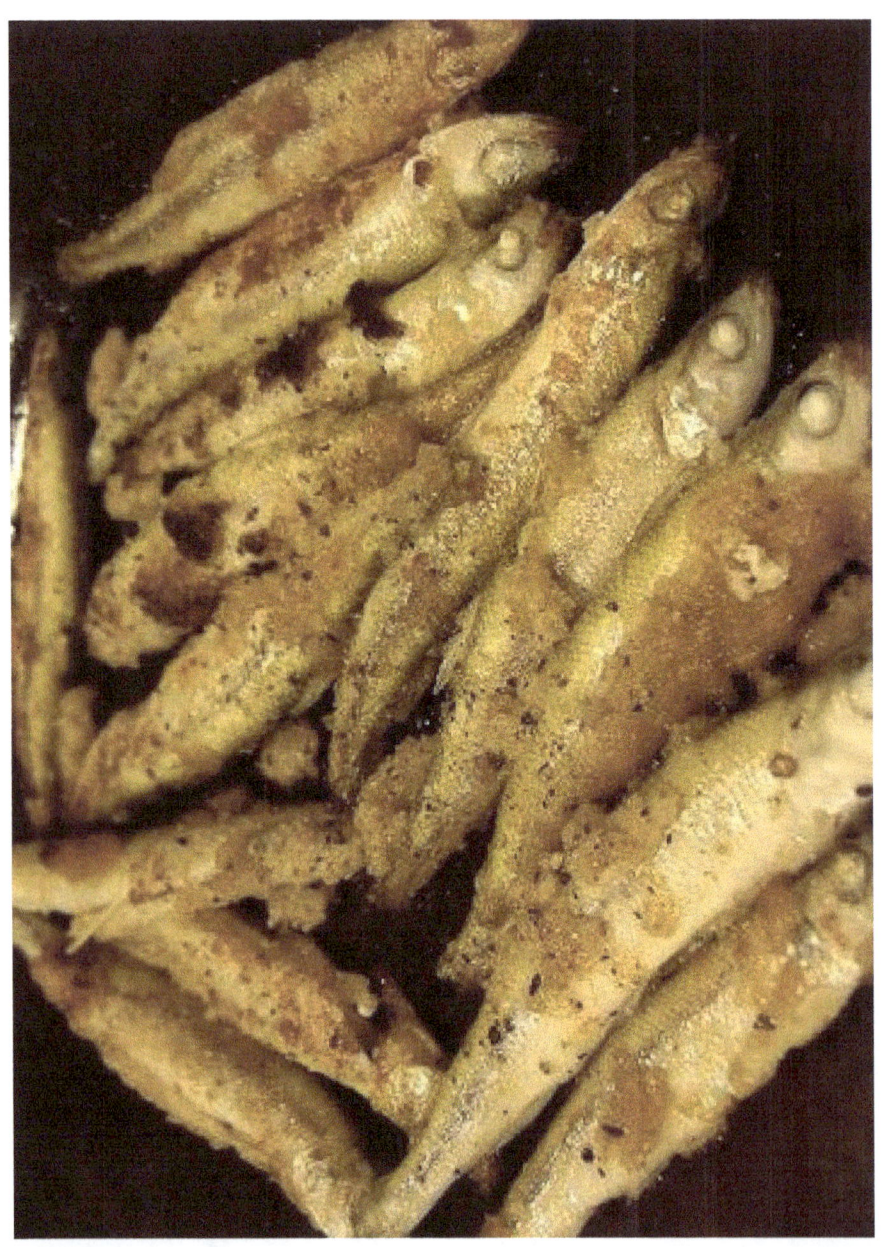

© copyright 2021 – all rights reserved.

the content contained within this book may not be reproduced, duplicated or transmitted without direct written permission from the author or the publisher.

under no circumstances will any blame or legal responsibility be held against the publisher, or author, for any damages, reparation, or monetary loss due to the information contained within this book. either directly or indirectly.

legal notice:

this book is copyright protected. this book is only for personal use. you cannot amend, distribute, sell, use, quote or paraphrase any part, or the content within this book, without the consent of the author or publisher.

disclaimer notice:

please note the information contained within this document is for educational and entertainment purposes only. all effort has been executed to present accurate, up to date, and reliable, complete information. no warranties of any kind are declared or implied. readers acknowledge that the author is not engaging in the rendering of legal, financial, medical or professional advice. the content within this book has been derived from various sources. please consult a licensed professional before attempting any techniques outlined in this book.

by reading this document, the reader agrees that under no circumstances is the author responsible for any losses, direct or indirect, which are incurred as a result of the use of information contained within this document, including, but not limited to, — errors, omissions, or inaccuracies.

Table of Contents

- CHEESE BURGER PATTIES 6
- GRILLED CHEESE CORN 8
- EGGPLANT FRIES 10
- AIR-FRIED ASPARAGUS 12
- BAKED POTATOES 14
- SCALLOPS AND DILL 16

BREAKFAST RECIPES 18
- LEAN LAMB AND TURKEY MEATBALLS WITH YOGURT 18
- EGGS 20
- CINNAMON PANCAKE 22
- SPINACH AND MUSHROOMS OMELET 24
- ALL BERRIES PANCAKES 26
- AUBERGINE AND TOMATO 28

SNACKS AND APPETIZER RECIPES 30
- CHEESY GARLIC BREAD 30
- MIXED AIR-FRIED VEGGIES 33
- PLANTAINS IN COCONUT SAUCE 36
- BEEF AND MANGO SKEWERS 38
- KALE CHIPS WITH LEMON YOGURT SAUCE 40
- BASIL PESTO BRUSCHETTA 42
- CINNAMON PEAR CHIPS 44

PORK, BEEF AND LAMB RECIPES 46
- AIR FRIED MEATLOAF 46
- PORK TENDERLOIN 48
- PORK BONDIOLA CHOP 49
- STEAK 51
- MARINATED LOIN POTATOES 53
- BEEF WITH MUSHROOMS 55
- CHEESY AND CRUNCHY RUSSIAN STEAKS 57

FISH & SEAFOOD RECIPES 59
BASIL-PARMESAN CRUSTED SALMON 59
CAJUN SHRIMP IN AIR FRYER 61
CRISPY AIR FRYER FISH 63
AIR FRYER LEMON COD 65

POULTRY RECIPES 67
CHICKEN TENDERS AND VEGETABLES 67
GREEK CHICKEN KEBABS 69
TANDOORI CHICKEN 71
HONEY LEMON GARLIC CHICKEN 73
BAKED LEMON PEPPER CHICKEN DRUMSTICKS 75
BALSAMIC GLAZED CHICKEN 77

VEGETABLES AND SIDES RECIPES 79
ROASTED PEANUT BUTTER SQUASH 79
ROASTED CHICKPEAS 81
CABBAGE WEDGES 83
BUFFALO CAULIFLOWER WINGS 85
SWEET POTATO CAULIFLOWER PATTIES 87
OKRA 89
CREAMED SPINACH 91
CHEESY EGGPLANT 93
CAULIFLOWER RICE 96

DESSERT RECIPES 99
COCOA CAKE 99
APPLE BREAD 101
BANANA BREAD 103
MINI LAVA CAKES 105
CRISPY APPLES 107

CHEESE BURGER PATTIES

Preparation Time: 5 minutes

Cooking Time: 16 minutes

Servings: 6

Nutritional values:

- Calories: 253 kcal
- Fat: 14 g
- Carbohydrates: 0.4 g
- Proteins: 29 g

Ingredients:

- 1 lb. ground beef
- 6 cheddar cheese slices
- Pepper and salt

Directions:

1. Adjust the temperature of the air fryer to 390°F.
2. Season your beef with salt and pepper.

3. Make six round-shaped patties from the mixture and place them into the air fryer basket.
4. Air fry the patties for 10 minutes.
5. Open the air fryer basket and place cheese slices on top of patties and place them into the air fryer with an additional cook time of 1 minute.

GRILLED CHEESE CORN

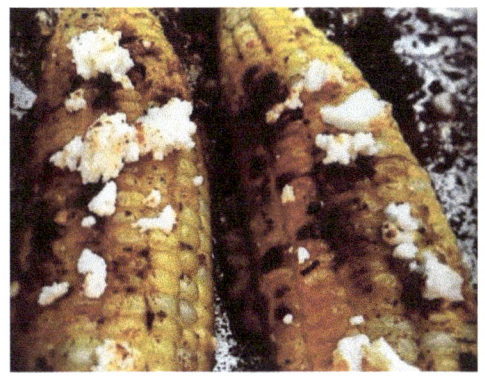

Preparation Time: 5 minutes

Cooking Time: 16 minutes

Servings: 2

Nutritional values:

- Calories: 150 kcal
- Fat: 10 g
- Carbohydrates: 7 g
- Proteins: 7 g

Ingredients:

- 2 whole corn on the cob, peel husks and discard silk
- 1 tsp. olive oil
- 2 tsps. Paprika
- ½ cup grated feta cheese

Directions:

1. Rub the olive oil over corn, then sprinkle with paprika and rub it all over the corn.
2. Adjust the temperature of the air fryer to 300°F.
3. Place the seasoned corn on the grill for 15-minutes.
4. Place corn on a serving dish, then sprinkles with grated cheese over corn. Serve.

EGGPLANT FRIES

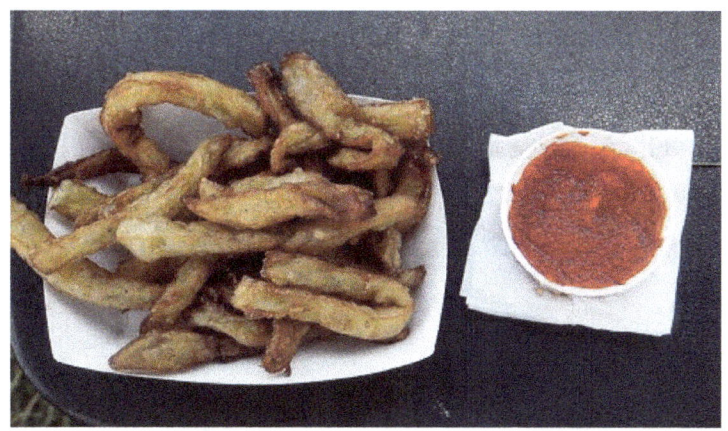

Preparation Time: 5 minutes

Cooking Time: 21 minutes

Servings: 4

Nutritional values:

- Calories: 113.2 kcal
- Fat: 7.2 g
- Carbohydrates: 12.3 g
- Proteins: 1.9 g

Ingredients:

- 1 eggplant, cut into 3-inch pieces
- ¼ cup water
- 1 tbsp. olive oil
- 4 tbsp. cornstarch
- Sea salt

Directions:

1. Adjust the temperature of the air fryer to 390°F.
2. Mix the eggplant, water, oil, and cornstarch in a bowl.
3. Place the eggplant fries in the air fryer basket and air fry them for 20 minutes. Serve warm.

AIR-FRIED ASPARAGUS

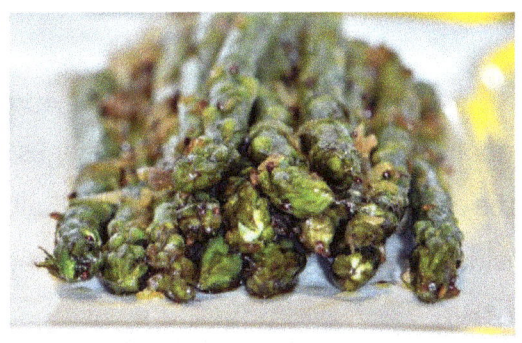

Preparation Time: 5 minutes

Cooking Time: 11 minutes

Servings: 4

Nutritional values:

- Calories: 118.2 kcal
- Fat: 8.1 g
- Carbohydrates: 10.3 g
- Proteins: 5.2 g

Ingredients:

- ½ bunch asparagus, trim off the bottoms
- Olive oil
- Salt

- Black pepper, ground

Directions:

1. In your air-fryer basket, add in the asparagus spears. Spray with the olive oil. Season with pepper and salt.
2. Set inside air-fryer and allow to bake for about 10 minutes at 400°F.
3. Serve and enjoy.

BAKED POTATOES

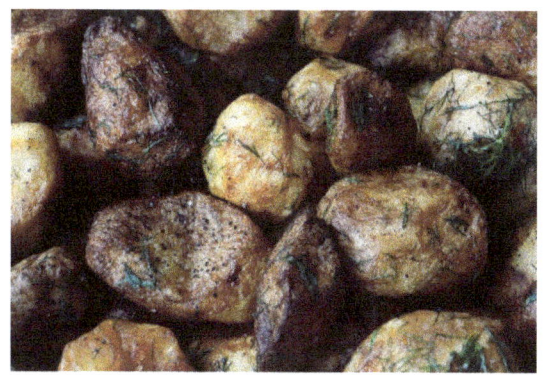

Preparation Time: 4 minutes

Cooking Time: 42 minutes

Servings: 3

Nutritional values:

- Calories: 110
- Fat: 0 g
- Carbohydrates: 26 g
- Proteins: 3 g

Ingredients:

- 3 medium-sized, scrubbed and rinsed russet potatoes
- Cooking spray
- ½ tsp. sea salt
- ½ tsp. garlic powder

Directions:

1. Place your potatoes in the Air Fryer basket, and spray with cooking spray on both sides. Sprinkle sea salt and garlic on all sides, rotating the potatoes as you got.
2. Use your hands to rub the potatoes to make sure everything becomes evenly coated.
3. Cook in the Air Fryer at 400°F for about 40 minutes, until fork-tender. Serve.

SCALLOPS AND DILL

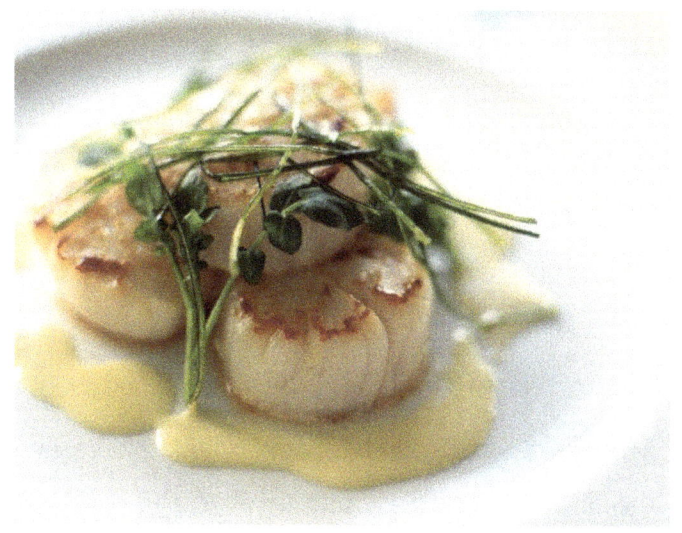

Preparation Time: 5 minutes

Cooking Time: 5 minutes

Servings: 4

Nutritional values:

- Calories: 451 kcal
- Carbohydrates: 3 g
- Fat: 39 g
- Proteins: 19 g

Ingredients:

- 1 lb. sea scallops
- 1 tbsp. lemon juice
- 1 tsp. dill
- 2 tsp. olive oil
- Black pepper and salt

Directions:

1. Mix scallops with oil, dill, pepper, lemon juice, and salt in the air fryer. Cook for 5 minutes at 360°F.
2. Dispose uncovered ones. Divide dill sauce and scallops on plates. Serve.

BREAKFAST RECIPES

LEAN LAMB AND TURKEY MEATBALLS WITH YOGURT

Preparation Time: 11 minutes

Cooking Time: 13 minutes

Servings: 4

Nutritional values:

- Calories: 154 kcal
- Fat: 2.5 g
- Carbohydrates: 9 g
- Proteins: 8.6 g

Ingredients:

- 1 egg white
- 4 ounces ground lean turkey
- 1 pound ground lean lamb

- 1 tsp. each cayenne pepper, ground coriander, red chili paste, salt, and ground cumin
- 2 garlic cloves, minced
- 1 ½ tbsp. parsley, chopped
- 1 tbsp. mint, chopped
- ¼ cup olive oil
- For the yogurt:
- 2 tbsp. buttermilk
- 1 garlic clove, minced
- ¼ cup mint, chopped
- ½ cup Greek yogurt, non-fat
- Salt to taste

Directions:

1. Set the Air Fryer to 390°F.
2. Mix all the ingredients for the meatballs in a bowl. Roll and mold them into golf-size round pieces. Arrange in the cooking basket. Cook for 8 minutes.
3. While waiting, combine all the ingredients for the mint yogurt in a bowl. Mix well.
4. Serve the meatballs with mint yogurt. Top with olives and fresh mint.

EGGS

Preparation Time: 9 minutes

Cooking Time: 18 minutes

Servings: 4

Nutritional values:

- Calories: 106 kcal
- Fat: 3.2 g
- Carbohydrates: 10 g
- Proteins: 9.0 g

Ingredients:

- 4 eggs
- 2 cups baby spinach, rinsed
- 1 tbsp. extra-virgin olive oil
- ½ cup cheddar cheese, reduced-fat, shredded, divided
- Pinch salt
- Pinch pepper

Directions:

1. Preheat the Air Fryer to 350°F.
2. Heat oil in a pan over medium-high flame. Cook the spinach until wilted. Drain the excess liquid. Put the cooked spinach into 4 greased ramekins.
3. Add a slice of bacon to each ramekin, crack an egg and put cheese on top. Season with salt and pepper.
4. Put the ramekins inside the cooking basket of the Air Fryer.
5. Cook for 15 minutes.

CINNAMON PANCAKE

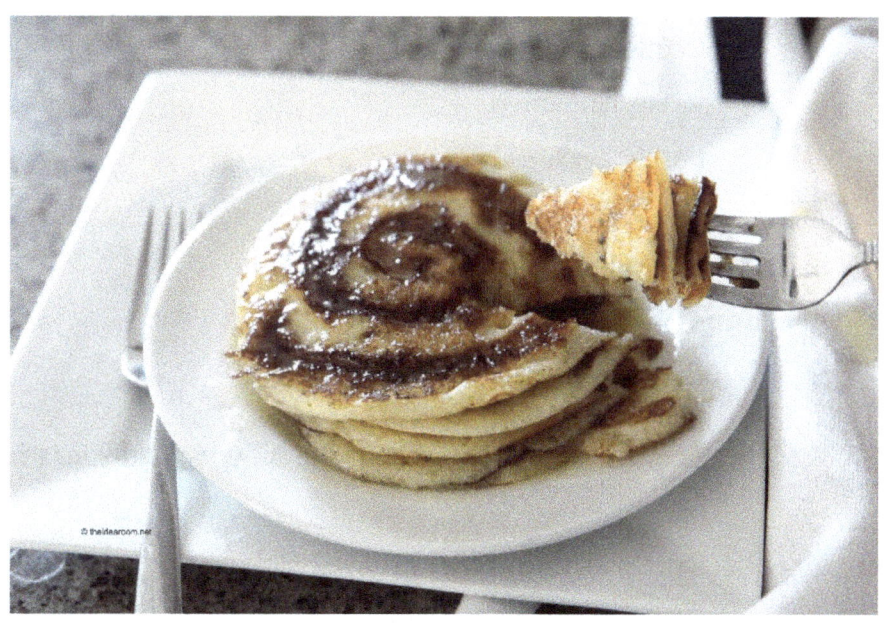

Preparation Time: 5 minutes

Cooking Time: 19 minutes

Servings: 4

Nutritional values:

- Calories: 106 kcal
- Fat: 3.2 g
- Carbohydrates: 10 g
- Proteins: 9.0 g

Ingredients:

- 2 eggs
- 2 cups cream cheese, reduced-fat
- ½ tsp. cinnamon
- 1 pack Stevia

Directions:

1. Preheat Air Fryer to 330°F.
2. Combine cream cheese, cinnamon, eggs, and stevia in a blender.
3. Pour ¼ of the mixture in the air fryer basket.
4. Cook for 2 minutes on each side.
5. Repeat the process with the rest of the mixture. Serve.

SPINACH AND MUSHROOMS OMELET

Preparation Time: 11 minutes

Cooking Time: 10-15 minutes

Servings: 4

Nutritional values:

- Calories: 110 kcal
- Fat: 1.3 g
- Carbohydrates: 9 g
- Proteins: 5.4 g

Ingredients:

- ½ cup spinach leaves
- 1 cup mushrooms
- 3 green onions
- 1 cup water
- ½ tsp. turmeric
- ½ red bell pepper

- 2 tbsp. butter, low fat
- 1 cup almond flour
- ½ tsp. onion powder
- ½ tsp. garlic powder
- ½ tsp. fresh ground black pepper
- ¼ tsp. ground thyme
- 2 tbsp. extra virgin olive oil
- 1 tsp. black salt
- Salsa, store-bought

Directions:

1. Preheat the Air Fryer to 300°F.
2. Rinse spinach leaves over tap water. Set aside.
3. In a mixing bowl, combine green onions, onion powder, garlic powder, red bell pepper, mushrooms, turmeric, thyme, olive oil, salt, and pepper. Mix well.
4. In another bowl, combine water and flour to form a smooth paste.
5. In a pan, heat olive oil. Sauté peppers and mushrooms for 3 minutes. Tip in spinach and cook for 3 minutes. Set aside.
6. In the Air fryer basket, pour omelet batter. Cook for 3 minutes before flipping. Place vegetables on top. Season with salt. Serve with salsa on the side.

ALL BERRIES PANCAKES

Preparation Time: 5 minutes

Cooking Time: 20 minutes

Servings: 4

Nutritional values:

- Calories: 57 kcal
- Fat: 0.3 g
- Carbohydrates: 14 g
- Proteins: 0.7 g

Ingredients:

- ½ cup frozen blueberries, thawed
- ½ cup frozen cranberries, thawed
- 1 cup coconut milk
- 2 tbsp. coconut oil for greasing
- 2 tbsp. stevia
- 1 cup whole wheat flour, finely milled
- 1 tbsp. baking powder

- 1 tsp. vanilla extract
- ¼ tsp. salt

Directions:

1. Preheat Air Fryer to 330°F.
2. In a mixing bowl, combine coconut oil, coconut milk, flour, stevia, baking powder, vanilla extract, and salt.
3. Gently fold in berries. Divide batter into equal portions. Pour into the Air fryer basket. Flip once the edges are set. Do not press down on pancakes.
4. Transfer to a plate. Sprinkle palm sugar. Serve.

AUBERGINE AND TOMATO

Preparation Time: 6 minutes

Cooking Time: 14 minutes

Servings: 2

Nutritional values:

- Calories: 140.3 kcal
- Fat: 3.4 g
- Carbohydrates: 26.6 g
- Proteins: 4.2 g

Ingredients:

- 1 aubergine, sliced thickly into 4 disks
- 1 tomato, sliced into 2 thick disks
- 2 tsp. feta cheese, reduced fat
- 2 fresh basil leaves, minced
- 2 balls, small buffalo mozzarella, reduced-fat, roughly torn
- Pinch salt
- Pinch black pepper

Directions:

1. Preheat Air Fryer to 330°F.
2. Spray a small amount of oil into the air fryer basket. Fry aubergine slices for 5 minutes or until golden brown on both sides. Transfer to a plate.
3. Fry tomato slices in batches for 5 minutes or until seared on both sides.
4. To serve, stack salad starting with an aubergine base, buffalo mozzarella, basil leaves, tomato slice, and ½ tsp. feta cheese.
5. Top with another slice of aubergine and ½ tsp. feta cheese. Serve.

SNACKS AND APPETIZER RECIPES

CHEESY GARLIC BREAD

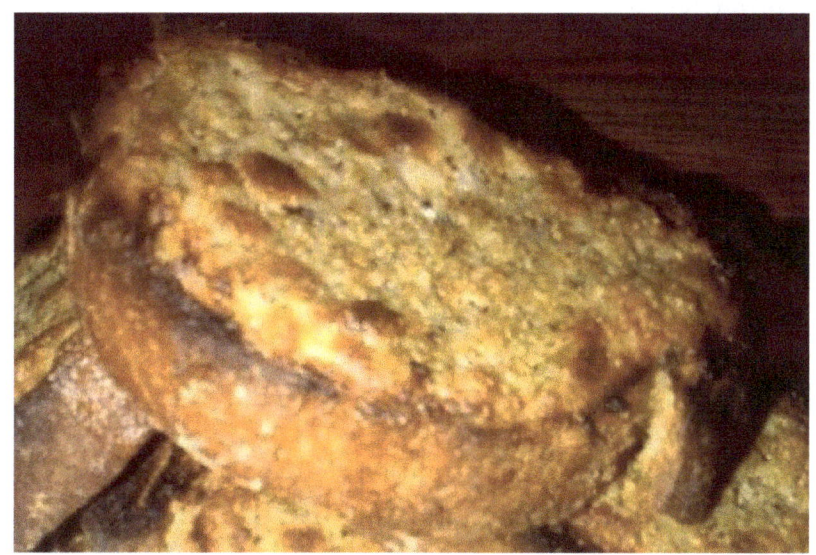

Preparation Time: 10 minutes

Cooking Time: 10 minutes

Servings: 8

Nutritional values:

- Calories: 209 kcal
- Fat: 8 g

- Carbohydrates: 29 g
- Proteins: 2.9 g

Ingredients:

- Fried garlic bread
- 1 medium baguette, halved lengthwise, cut sides toasted
- 2 garlic cloves, whole
- 4 tbsp. extra virgin olive oil
- 2 tbsp. fresh parsley, minced

Blue cheese dip:

- 1 tbsp. fresh parsley, minced
- ¼ cup fresh chives, minced
- ¼ tsp. Tabasco sauce
- 1 tbsp. lemon juice, freshly squeezed
- ½ cup Greek yogurt, low fat
- ¼ cup blue cheese, reduced fat
- 1/16 tsp. salt
- 1/16 tsp. white pepper

Directions:

1. Preheat machine to 400°F.
2. Mix oil and parsley in a small bowl.

3. Vigorously rub garlic cloves on cut/toasted sides of the baguette. Dispose of garlic nubs.
4. Using a pastry brush, spread parsley-infused oil on the cut side of the bread.
5. Place the bread cut-side down on a chopping board. Slice into inch-thick half-moons.
6. Place bread slices in an Air Fryer basket. Fry for 3 to 5 minutes or until bread browns a little. Shake contents of the basket once midway through. Place cooked pieces on a serving platter. Repeat the step for the remaining bread.
7. To prepare blue cheese dip: mix all the ingredients in a bowl.
8. Place equal portions of fried bread on plates. Serve with blue cheese dip on the side.

MIXED AIR-FRIED VEGGIES

Preparation Time: 10 minutes

Cooking Time: 10 minutes

Servings: 4

Nutritional values:

- Calories: 109 kcal
- Fat: 2.6 g
- Carbohydrates: 4.0 g
- Proteins: 2.9 g

Ingredients:

- Oil for spraying

Dip:

- 1 avocado, pitted, peeled, flesh scooped out
- 4 oz. of feta cheese, reduced fat
- 2 leeks, minced
- 1 lime, freshly squeezed
- ¼ cup fresh parsley, chopped roughly

- 1/16 tsp. black pepper
- 1/16 tsp. salt

Vegetables:

- 1 zucchini, sliced into matchsticks
- 1 carrot, sliced into matchsticks
- 1 cup panko breadcrumbs. Add more if needed
- 1 parsnip, sliced into matchsticks
- 1 large egg, whisked, add more if needed
- 1 cup all-purpose flour, add more if needed
- 1/8 tsp. flaky sea salt

Directions:

1. Preheat the Air Fryer to 400°F.
2. Season carrots, parsnips, and zucchini with salt.
3. Dredge carrots with flour first, then dip them into the whisked egg, and finally into breadcrumbs. Place breaded pieces on a baking sheet lined with parchment paper. Repeat the step for all the carrots. Then do the same for the parsnips and the zucchini.
4. Lightly spray vegetables with oil. Place a generous handful of carrots in the Air Fryer basket. Fry for 10 minutes or until breading turns golden brown, shaking contents of the basket once midway. Place cooked pieces on a plate. Repeat the step for the remaining carrots.

5. Do the earlier step for parsnips and then zucchini.
6. For the dip, except for salt, place the remaining ingredients in a food processor. Pulse a couple of times, and then process to the desired consistency scraping the down sides of the machine often. Taste. Add salt only if needed. Place in an airtight container. Chill until needed.
7. Place equal portions of cooked vegetables on plates. Serve with a small amount of avocado-feta dip on the side.

PLANTAINS IN COCONUT SAUCE

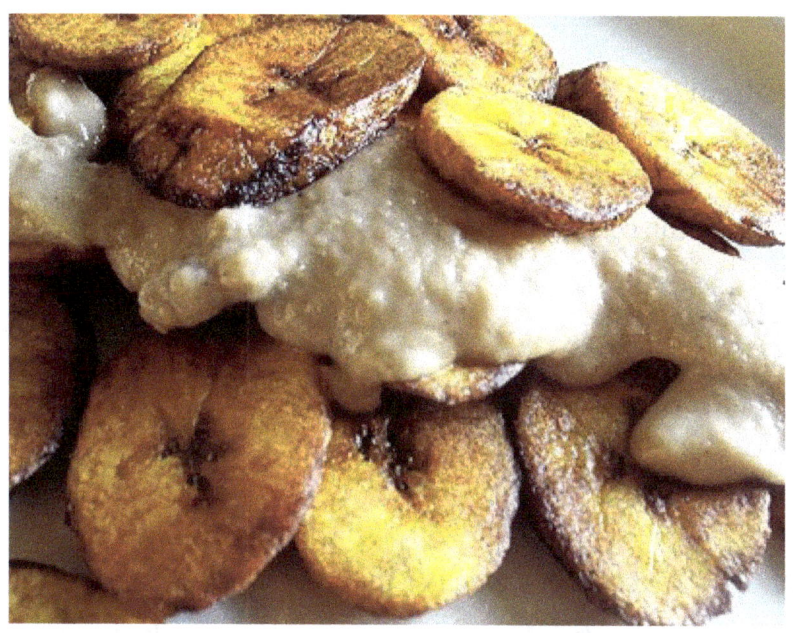

Preparation Time: 10 minutes

Cooking Time: 10 minutes

Servings: 8

Nutritional values:

- Calories: 236 kcal

- Fat: 1.5 g
- Carbohydrates: 0 g
- Proteins: 1 g

Ingredients:

- 6 ripe plantains, peeled, quartered lengthwise
- 1 can coconut cream
- 1 tbsp. Splenda

Directions:

1. Preheat the Air Fryer to 330F.
2. Pour coconut cream in a thick-bottomed saucepan set over high heat; bring to boil. Reduce heat to lowest setting; simmer uncovered until the cream is reduced by half and darkens in color. Turn off heat.
3. Whisk in honey until smooth. Cool completely before using. Lightly grease a non-stick skillet with coconut oil.
4. Layer plantains in the Air Fryer basket and fry until golden on both sides; drain on paper towels. Place plantain into plates.
5. Drizzle in a small amount of coconut sauce. Serve.

BEEF AND MANGO SKEWERS

Preparation Time: 10 minutes

Cooking Time: 4–7 minutes

Servings: 4

Nutritional values:

- Calories: 245 kcal
- Fat: 9 g
- Carbohydrates: 15 g
- Proteins: 26 g

Ingredients:

- ¾ pound (340 g) of beef sirloin tip, cut into 1-inch cubes
- 2 tbsp. balsamic vinegar
- 1 tbsp. olive oil
- 1 tbsp. honey
- ½ tsp. dried marjoram
- Pinch salt
- Freshly ground black pepper, to taste
- 1 mango

Directions:

1. Put the beef cubes in a medium bowl and add the balsamic vinegar, olive oil, honey, marjoram, salt, and pepper. Mix well, then rub the marinade into the beef with your hands. Set aside.
2. To prepare the mango, stand it on end and cut the skin off using a sharp knife. Then carefully cut around the oval pit to remove the flesh. Cut the mango into 1-inch cubes.
3. Thread metal skewers alternating with three beef cubes and two mango cubes. Place the skewers in the Air Fryer basket.
4. Air fry at 390°F (199°C) for 4 to 7 minutes or until the beef is browned and at least 145°F (63°C).

KALE CHIPS WITH LEMON YOGURT SAUCE

Preparation Time: 10 minutes

Cooking Time: 5 minutes

Servings: 4

Nutritional values:

- Calories: 155 kcal
- Fat: 8 g
- Carbohydrates: 13 g
- Proteins: 8 g

Ingredients:

- 1 cup plain Greek yogurt
- 3 tbsp. freshly squeezed lemon juice
- 2 tbsp. honey mustard
- ½ tsp. dried oregano
- 1 bunch curly kale
- 2 tbsp. olive oil

- ½ tsp. salt
- 1/8 tsp. pepper

Directions:

1. In a small bowl, mix the yogurt, lemon juice, honey mustard, and oregano, and set aside.
2. Remove the stems and ribs from the kale with a sharp knife. Cut the leaves into 2- to 3-inch pieces.
3. Toss the kale with olive oil, salt, and pepper. Rub the oil into the leaves with your hands.
4. Air fry the kale in batches at 390°F (199°C) until crisp, about 5 minutes, shaking the basket once during cooking time. Serve with the yogurt sauce.

BASIL PESTO BRUSCHETTA

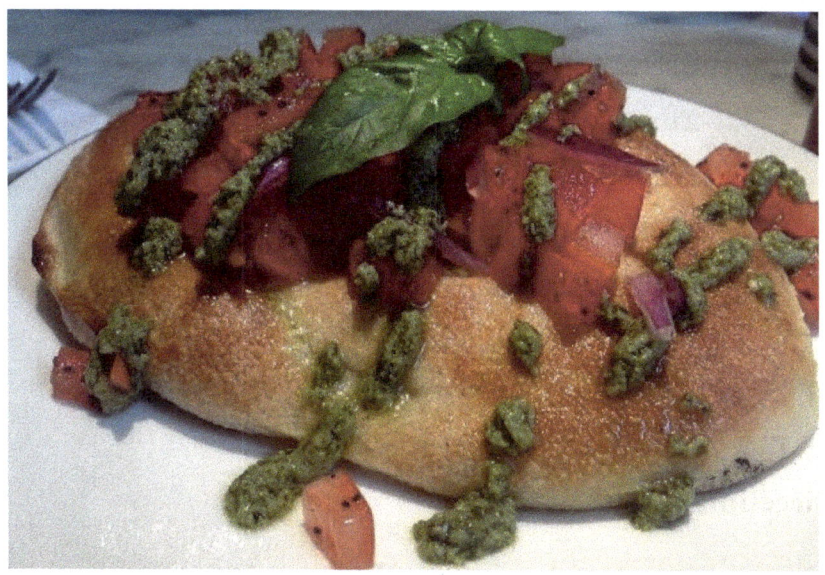

Preparation Time: 10 minutes

Cooking Time: 4–8 minutes

Servings: 4

Nutritional values:

- Calories: 463
- Fat: 25 g
- Carbohydrates: 41 g
- Proteins: 19 g

Ingredients:

- 8 slices French bread, ½ inch thick
- 2 tbsp. softened butter
- 1 cup shredded Mozzarella cheese
- ½ cup basil pesto
- 1 cup chopped grape tomatoes
- 2 green onions, thinly sliced

Directions:

1. Spread the bread with the butter and place butter-side up in the Air Fryer basket. Bake at 350°F (177°C) for 3 to 5 minutes or until the bread is light golden brown.
2. Remove the bread from the basket and top each piece with some of the cheese. Return to the basket in batches and bake until the cheese melts, about 1 to 3 minutes.
3. Meanwhile, combine the pesto, tomatoes, and green onions in a small bowl.
4. When the cheese has melted, remove the bread from the Air Fryer and place on a serving plate. Top each slice with some of the pesto mixtures and serve.

CINNAMON PEAR CHIPS

Preparation Time: 15 minutes

Cooking Time: 9–13 minutes

Servings: 4

Nutritional values:

- Calories: 31 kcal
- Fat: 0 g
- Carbohydrates: 8 g
- Proteins: 7 g

Ingredients:

- 2 firm Bosc pears, cut crosswise into 1/8-inch-thick slices
- 1 tbsp. freshly squeezed lemon juice
- ½ tsp. ground cinnamon
- 1/8 tsp. ground cardamom or ground nutmeg

Directions:

1. Separate the smaller stem-end pear rounds from the larger rounds with seeds. Remove the core and seeds from the larger slices. Sprinkle all slices with lemon juice, cinnamon, and cardamom.
2. Put the smaller chips into the Air Fryer basket. Air fry at 380°F (193°C) for 3 to 5 minutes, until light golden brown, shaking the basket once during cooking. Remove from the Air Fryer.
3. Repeat with the larger slices, air frying for 6 to 8 minutes, until light golden brown, shaking the basket once during cooking.
4. Remove the chips from the Air Fryer. Cool and serve or store in an airtight container at room temperature for up to 2 days.

PORK, BEEF AND LAMB RECIPES

AIR FRIED MEATLOAF

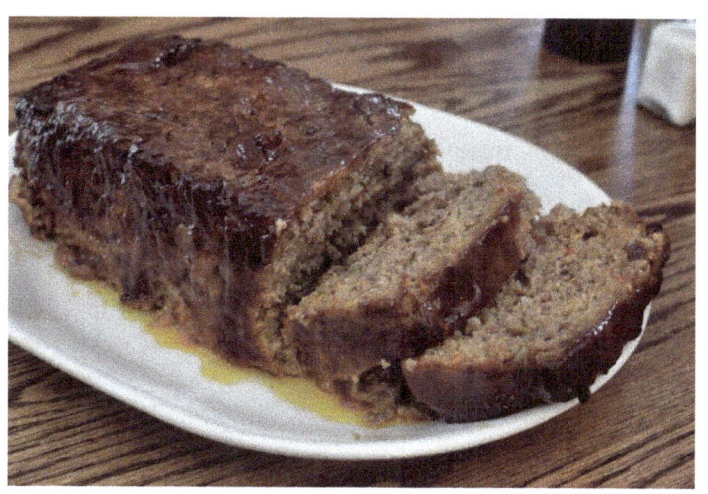

Preparation Time: 6 minutes

Cooking Time: 25-30 minutes

Servings: 2

Nutritional values:

- Calories: 381 kcal
- Fat: 5 g
- Carbohydrates: 9.6 g
- Proteins: 38 g

Ingredients:

- ½ lb. ground beef
- ½ lb. ground turkey
- 1 onion, chopped
- ¼ cup panko bread crumbs
- 3 tbsp. ketchup
- ¼ cup brown sugar
- 1 egg, beaten
- Salt and pepper to taste

Directions:

1. Preheat the air fryer to 400°F.
2. Let the ground beef and ground turkey sit on the counter for 10 to 15 minutes, as it will be easier to hand mix without being chilled from the refrigerator.
3. Combine all the ingredients.
4. Form into a loaf in a dish and place the dish in the frying basket. Spritz the top with a little olive oil.
5. Bake for 25 minutes, or until well browned. Let settle for about 10 minutes before serving.

PORK TENDERLOIN

Preparation Time: 9 minutes

Cooking Time: 33 minutes

Servings: 6

Nutritional values:

- Calories: 419 kcal
- Fat: 3.5 g
- Carbohydrates: 0 g
- Proteins: 26 g

Ingredients:

- 1-½ lbs. pork tenderloin

Directions:

1. Adjust the temperature of the Air Fryer to 370°F.
2. Lay the pork in the Air Fryer basket.
3. Cook at 400°F for about 30 minutes, turning halfway through cooking time for a proper cook.
4. Serve.

PORK BONDIOLA CHOP

Preparation Time: 8 minutes

Cooking Time: 22 minutes

Servings: 4

Nutritional values:

- Calories: 265 kcal
- Fat: 20.36 g
- Carbohydrates: 0 g
- Proteins: 19.14 g

Ingredients:

- 1 kg bondiola in pieces
- Breadcrumbs
- 2 beaten eggs
- Seasoning to taste

Directions:

1. Cut the bondiola into small pieces

2. Add seasonings to taste.
3. Pour the beaten eggs on the seasoned bondiola.
4. Add the breadcrumbs.
5. Cook in the air fryer for 20 minutes while turning the food halfway.
6. Serve

STEAK

Preparation Time: 6 minutes

Cooking Time: 18 minutes

Servings: 2

Nutritional values:

- Calories: 82 kcal
- Fat: 5 g
- Carbohydrates: 0 g
- Proteins: 8.7 g

Ingredients:

- 2 steaks, grass-fed, each about 6 ounces and ¾ inch thick
- 1 tbsp. butter, unsalted
- ¾ tsp. ground black pepper
- ½ tsp. garlic powder
- ¾ tsp. salt
- 1 tsp. olive oil

Directions:

1. Switch on the air fryer, insert fryer basket, grease it with olive oil, then shut with its lid, set the fryer at 400°F, and preheat for 5 minutes.
2. Meanwhile, coat the steaks with oil and then season with black pepper, garlic, and salt.
3. Open the fryer, add steaks in it, close with its lid and cook 10 to 18 minutes at until nicely golden and steaks are cooked to desired doneness, flipping the steaks halfway through the frying.
4. When the air fryer beeps, open its lid and transfer steaks to a cutting board.
5. Take two large aluminum foil pieces, place a steak on each piece, top steak with ½ tbsp. butter, then cover with foil and let it rest for 5 minutes.
6. Serve straight away.

MARINATED LOIN POTATOES

Preparation Time: 8 minutes

Cooking Time: 40-50 minutes

Servings: 2

Nutritional values:

- Calories: 136 kcal
- Fat: 5.1 g
- Carbohydrates: 1.9 g
- Proteins: 20.7 g

Ingredients:

- 2 medium potatoes
- 4 fillets marinated loin
- A little extra virgin olive oil
- Salt

Directions:

1. Peel the potatoes and cut. Cut with match-sized mandolin, potatoes with a cane but very thin.
2. Wash and immerse in water for 30 minutes.
3. Drain and dry well.
4. Add a little oil and stir so that the oil permeates well in all the potatoes.
5. Go to the basket of the air fryer and distribute well.
6. Cook at 160°C for 10 minutes.
7. Take out the basket, shake so that the potatoes take off. Let the potato tender. If it is not, leave 5 more minutes.
8. Place the steaks on top of the potatoes.
9. Select 10 minutes, and 180°C for 5 minutes again.

BEEF WITH MUSHROOMS

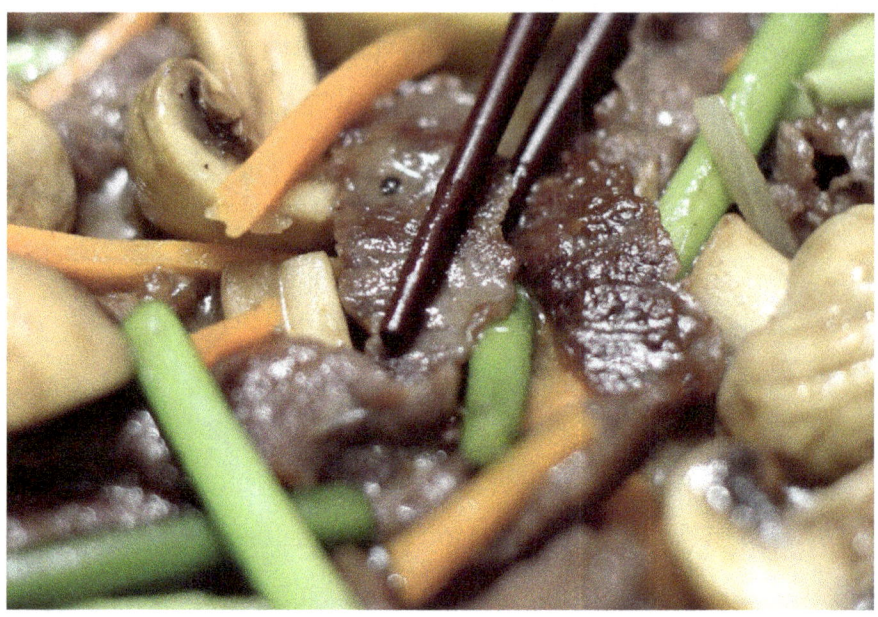

Preparation Time: 8 minutes

Cooking Time: 41 minutes

Servings: 4

Nutritional values:

- Calories: 175
- Fat: 6.2 g

- Carbohydrates: 4.4 g
- Proteins: 24.9 g

Ingredients:

- 300 g beef
- 150 g mushrooms
- 1 onion
- 1 tsp. olive oil
- 100 g vegetable broth
- 1 tsp. basil
- 1 tsp. chili
- 30 g tomato juice

Directions:

1. For this recipe, you should take a solid piece of beef. Take the beef and pierce the meat with a knife.
2. Rub it with olive oil, basil, chili, and lemon juice.
3. Chop the onion and mushrooms and pour it with vegetable broth.
4. Cook the vegetables for 5 minutes.
5. Take a big tray and put the meat in it. Add vegetable broth to the tray too. It will make the meat juicy.
6. Preheat the air fryer oven to 180°C and cook it for 35 minutes.

CHEESY AND CRUNCHY RUSSIAN STEAKS

Preparation Time: 6 minutes

Cooking Time: 22 minutes

Servings: 4

Nutritional values:

- Calories: 123.2
- Fat: 3.41 g
- Carbohydrates: 0 g
- Proteins: 20.99 g

Ingredients:

- 800 g minced pork
- 200 g cream cheese
- 50g peeled walnuts
- 1 onion
- Salt
- Ground pepper

- 1 egg
- Breadcrumbs
- Extra virgin olive oil

Directions:

1. Put the onion cut into quarters in the Thermo mix glass and select 5 seconds speed 5.
2. Add the minced meat, cheese, egg, salt, and pepper.
3. Select 10 seconds, speed 5, turn left.
4. Add the chopped and peeled walnuts and select 4 seconds, turn left, speed 5.
5. Pass the dough to a bowl.
6. Make Russian steaks and go through breadcrumbs.
7. Paint the Russian fillets with extra virgin olive oil on both sides with a brush.
8. Put in the basket of the air fryer without stacking the Russian fillets.
9. Select 180°C for 15 minutes.

FISH & SEAFOOD RECIPES

BASIL-PARMESAN CRUSTED SALMON

Preparation Time: 5 minutes

Cooking Time: 16 minutes

Servings: 4

Nutritional values:

- Calories: 289
- Fat: 18.5 g
- Carbohydrates: 1.5 g
- Proteins: 30 g

Ingredients:

- Grated Parmesan: 3 tbsp.
- Skinless four salmon fillets
- Salt: ¼ tsp.
- Freshly ground black pepper

- Low-fat mayonnaise: 3 tbsp.
- Basil leaves, chopped
- Half lemon

Directions:

1. Let the air fryer preheat to 400°F. Spray the basket with olive oil.
2. With salt, pepper, and lemon juice, season the salmon.
3. In a bowl, mix two tbsp. of Parmesan cheese with mayonnaise and basil leaves.
4. Add this mix and more parmesan on top of salmon and cook for seven minutes or until fully cooked.
5. Serve hot.

CAJUN SHRIMP IN AIR FRYER

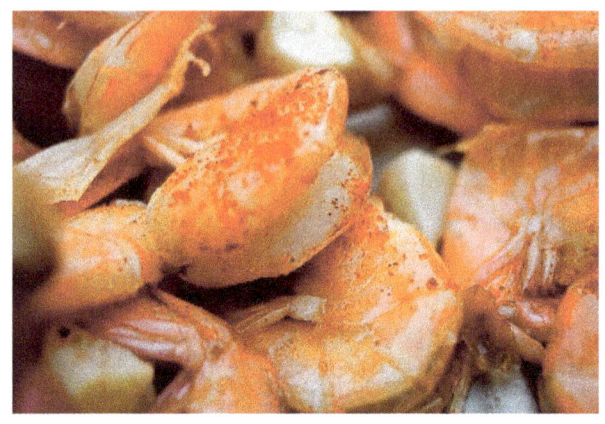

Preparation Time: 9 minutes

Cooking Time: 22 minutes

Servings: 4

Nutritional values:

- Calories: 284 kcal
- Fat: 14 g
- Carbohydrates: 8 g
- Proteins: 31 g

Ingredients:

- 24 extra-jumbo shrimp, peeled,
- 2 tbsp. olive oil
- 1 tbsp. Cajun seasoning
- 1 zucchini, thick slices (half-moons)
- ¼ cup cooked turkey
- 2 yellow squash, sliced half-moons
- Kosher salt: ¼ tsp.

Directions:

1. In a bowl, mix the shrimp with Cajun seasoning.
2. In another bowl, add zucchini, turkey, salt, squash, and coat with oil.
3. Let the air fryer preheat to 400°F
4. Move the shrimp and vegetable mix to the fryer basket and cook for three minutes.
5. Serve hot.

CRISPY AIR FRYER FISH

Preparation Time: 11 minutes

Cooking Time: 18 minutes

Servings: 4

Nutritional values:

- Calories: 254 kcal
- Fat: 12.7 g
- Carbohydrates: 8.2 g
- Proteins: 17.5 g

Ingredients:

- 2 tsp. Old bay
- 4–6, cut in half, whiting fish fillets
- ¾ cup fine cornmeal
- ¼ cup flour
- 1 tsp paprika
- 1/2 tsp. garlic powder:
- 1 ½ tsp. salt
- ½ freshly ground black pepper

Directions:

1. In a Ziplock bag, add all ingredients and coat the fish fillets with it.
2. Spray oil on the basket of the air fryer and put the fish in it.
3. Cook for ten minutes at 400°F. flip fish if necessary and coat with oil spray and cook for another seven-minute.
4. Serve with salad green.

AIR FRYER LEMON COD

Preparation Time: 5 minutes

Cooking Time: 18 minutes

Servings: 1

Nutritional values:

- Calories: 101 kcal
- Fat: 1 g
- Carbohydrates: 10 g
- Proteins: 16g

Ingredients:

- One cod fillet
- Dried parsley
- Kosher salt and pepper to taste
- Garlic powder
- One lemon

Directions:

1. In a bowl, mix all ingredients and coat the fish fillet with spices.
2. Slice the lemon and lay it at the bottom of the air fryer basket.
3. Put spiced fish on top. Cover the fish with lemon slices.
4. Cook for ten minutes at 375°F, the internal temperature of fish should be 145°F.
5. Serve.

POULTRY RECIPES

CHICKEN TENDERS AND VEGETABLES

Preparation Time: 9 minutes

Cooking Time: 18 minutes

Servings: 4

Nutritional values:

- Calories: 379 kcal
- Fat: 8 g
- Carbohydrates: 35 g
- Proteins: 41 g

Ingredients:

- 1 pound (454 g) chicken tenders
- 1 tbsp. honey
- Pinch salt
- Freshly ground black pepper, to taste

- ½ cup soft, fresh bread crumbs
- ½ tsp. dried thyme
- 1 tbsp. olive oil
- 2 carrots, sliced
- 12 small red potatoes

Directions:

1. In a medium bowl, toss the chicken tenders with honey, salt, and pepper.
2. In a shallow bowl, combine the bread crumbs, thyme, and olive oil, and mix.
3. Coat the tenders in the bread crumbs, pressing firmly onto the meat.
4. Place the carrots and potatoes in the air fryer basket and top with the chicken tenders.
5. Roast at 380°F (193°C) for 18 to 20 minutes or until the chicken is cooked to 165°F (74°C) and the vegetables are tender, shaking the basket halfway during the cooking time.

GREEK CHICKEN KEBABS

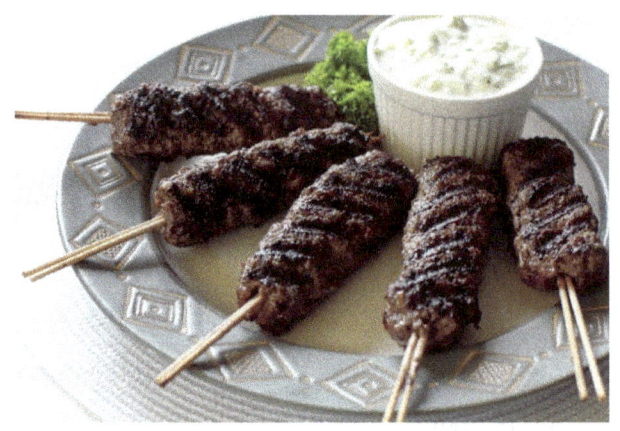

Preparation Time: 15 minutes

Cooking Time: 16 minutes

Servings: 4

Nutritional values:

- Calories: 164 kcal
- Fat: 4 g
- Carbohydrates: 4 g
- Proteins: 27 g

Ingredients:

- 3 tbsp. freshly squeezed lemon juice
- 2 tsp. olive oil
- 2 tbsp. chopped fresh flat-leaf parsley
- ½ tsp. dried oregano
- ½ tsp. dried mint
- 1 pound (454 g) low-sodium boneless, skinless chicken breasts, cut into 1-inch pieces
- 1 cup cherry tomatoes
- 1 small yellow summer squash, cut into 1-inch cubes

Directions:

1. In a large bowl, whisk the lemon juice, olive oil, parsley, oregano, and mint.
2. Add the chicken and stir to coat. Let stand for 10 minutes at room temperature.
3. Alternating the items, thread the chicken, tomatoes, and squash onto 8 bamboo or metal skewers that fit in an air fryer. Brush with marinade.
4. Air fry the kebabs at 380°F (193°C) for about 15 minutes, brushing once with any remaining marinade until the chicken reaches an internal temperature of 165°F (74°C) on a meat thermometer. Discard any remaining marinade. Serve immediately.

TANDOORI CHICKEN

Preparation Time: 5 minutes

Cooking Time: 15 minutes

Servings: 4

Nutritional values:

- Calories: 198 kcal
- Fat: 5 g
- Carbohydrates: 4 g
- Proteins: 33 g

Ingredients:

- 2/3 cup plain low-fat yogurt
- 2 tbsp. freshly squeezed lemon juice
- 2 tsp. curry powder
- ½ tsp. ground cinnamon
- 2 garlic cloves, minced
- 2 tsp. olive oil
- 4 (5-ounce / 142-g) low-sodium boneless, skinless chicken breasts

Directions:

1. In a medium bowl, whisk the yogurt, lemon juice, curry powder, cinnamon, garlic, and olive oil.
2. With a sharp knife, cut thin slashes into the chicken. Add it to the yogurt mixture and turn to coat. Let stand for 10 minutes at room temperature. You can also prepare this ahead of time and marinate the chicken in the refrigerator for up to 24 hours.
3. Remove the chicken from the marinade and shake off any excess liquid. Discard any remaining marinade.
4. Roast the chicken at 360°F (182°C) for 10 minutes. With tongs, carefully turn each piece. Roast for 8 to 13 minutes more, or until the chicken reaches an internal temperature of 165°F (74°C) on a meat thermometer. Serve immediately.

HONEY LEMON GARLIC CHICKEN

Preparation Time: 8 minutes

Cooking Time: 20 minutes

Servings: 4

Nutritional values:

- Calories: 214 kcal
- Fat: 4 g
- Carbohydrates: 10 g
- Proteins: 33 g

Ingredients:

- 4 (5-ounce / 142-g) low-sodium boneless, skinless chicken breasts, cut into 4-by-½-inch strips
- 2 tsp. olive oil
- 2 tbsp. cornstarch
- 3 garlic cloves, minced
- ½ cup low-sodium chicken broth

- ¼ cup freshly squeezed lemon juice
- 1 tbsp. honey
- ½ tsp. dried thyme
- Brown rice, cooked (optional)

Directions:

1. In a large bowl, mix the chicken and olive oil. Sprinkle with the cornstarch. Toss to coat.
2. Add the garlic and transfer to a baking pan. Bake in the air fryer at 400°F (204°C) for 10 minutes, stirring once during cooking.
3. Add the chicken broth, lemon juice, honey, and thyme to the chicken mixture. Bake for 6 to 9 minutes more, or until the sauce is slightly thickened and the chicken reaches an internal temperature of 165°F (74°C) on a meat thermometer. Serve over hot cooked brown rice, if desired.

BAKED LEMON PEPPER CHICKEN DRUMSTICKS

Preparation Time: 5 minutes

Cooking Time: 22 minutes

Servings: 4

Nutritional values:

- Calories: 195 kcal
- Fat: 11 g
- Carbohydrates: 1 g
- Proteins: 23 g

Ingredients:

- Olive oil spray
- 6 chicken drumsticks
- 1 tsp. lemon pepper
- ½ tsp. salt
- ½ tsp. granulated garlic
- ½ tsp. onion powder

Directions:

1. Spray the chicken with olive oil and spray the air fryer basket or line it with parchment paper.
2. In a small bowl, combine the lemon pepper, salt, garlic, and onion powder.
3. Place the chicken in the prepared air fryer basket, and sprinkle with half of the seasoning mixture.
4. Bake at 370°F (188°C) for 10 minutes.
5. Flip the drumsticks, and spray them with more olive oil and sprinkle with the remaining seasoning.
6. Place the chicken back in the air fryer, bake for an additional 12 minutes, and serve.
7. The chicken is done when the internal temperature reaches 180°F (82°C), and the juices run clear. It should look slightly crisp on the outside.

BALSAMIC GLAZED CHICKEN

Preparation Time: 5 minutes

Cooking Time: 22 minutes

Servings: 4

Nutritional values:

- Calories: 263 kcal
- Fat: 11 g
- Carbohydrates: 3 g
- Proteins: 38 g

Ingredients:

Glaze:

- 1 tbsp. olive oil
- 2 tsp. balsamic vinegar
- 1 tsp. minced garlic
- 1 tsp. honey
- ½ tsp. cornstarch
- ¼ tsp. salt
- ¼ tsp. ground black pepper

Chicken:

- Olive oil spray
- 4 bone-in chicken thighs
- 2 tsp. granulated garlic, divided
- 1 tsp. salt, divided
- ½ tsp. ground black pepper, divided
- ¼ tsp. onion powder, divided

Directions:

1. Make the Glaze
2. In a small bowl, whisk together the olive oil, balsamic vinegar, garlic, honey, cornstarch, salt, and pepper. Set aside.
3. Make the Chicken
4. Spray the chicken and the air fryer basket with olive oil.
5. Place the chicken in the air fryer basket, and sprinkle with about half of the garlic, salt, pepper, and onion powder.
6. Bake at 380°F (193°C) for 10 minutes.
7. Remove the chicken and flip the pieces. Spray it with more olive oil, and sprinkle with the remaining seasoning.
8. Place the chicken back in the air fryer and bake for an additional 10 minutes.
9. Remove the chicken, and brush with the prepared glaze. Bake for an additional 2 minutes, or until the sauce is sticky and caramelized, and serve.

VEGETABLES AND SIDES RECIPES

ROASTED PEANUT BUTTER SQUASH

Preparation Time: 5 minutes

Cooking Time: 22 minutes

Servings: 4

Nutritional values:

- Carbohydrates: 22 g
- Fat: 3 g
- Proteins: 1 g

Ingredients:

- 1 butternut squash, peeled
- 1 tsp. cinnamon
- 1 tbsp. olive oil

Directions:

1. Switch on the air fryer, insert fryer basket, grease it with olive oil, then shut with its lid, set the fryer at 220°F and preheat for 5 minutes.
2. Meanwhile, peel the squash 400, cut it into 1-inch pieces, and then place them in a bowl.
3. Drizzle oil over squash pieces, sprinkle with cinnamon, and then, toss until well coated.
4. Open the fryer, add squash pieces in it, close with its lid and cook for 17 minutes until nicely golden and crispy, shaking every 5 minutes.
5. When the air fryer beeps, open its lid, transfer squash onto a serving plate and serve.

ROASTED CHICKPEAS

Preparation Time: 35 minutes

Cooking Time: 25 minutes

Servings: 6

Nutritional values:

- Calories: 124 kcal
- Fat: 4.4 g
- Carbohydrates: 17.4 g
- Proteins: 4.7 g

Ingredients:

- 15-ounce cooked chickpeas
- 1 tsp. garlic powder
- 1 tbsp. Nutritional yeast
- 1/8 tsp. cumin
- 1 tsp. smoked paprika
- ½ tsp. salt
- 1 tbsp. olive oil

Directions:

1. Take a large baking sheet, line it with paper towels, spread chickpeas on it, cover the peas with paper towels, and rest for 30 minutes or until chickpeas are dried.
2. Then switch on the air fryer, insert fryer basket, grease it with olive oil, then shut with its lid, set the fryer at 355°F and preheat for 5 minutes.
3. Place dried chickpeas in a bowl, add remaining ingredients and toss until well coated.
4. Open the fryer, add chickpeas in it, close with its lid and cook for 20 minutes until nicely golden and crispy, shaking the chickpeas every 5 minutes.
5. When the air fryer beeps, open its lid, transfer chickpeas onto a serving bowl, and serve.

CABBAGE WEDGES

Preparation Time: 10 minutes

Cooking Time: 29 minutes

Servings: 6

Nutritional values:

- Calories: 123 kcal
- Fat: 11 g
- Carbohydrates: 2 g
- Proteins: 4 g

Ingredients:

- 1 small head green cabbage
- 6 strips of bacon, thick-cut, pastured
- 1 tsp. onion powder
- ½ tsp. ground black pepper
- 1 tsp. garlic powder
- ¾ tsp. salt
- ¼ tsp. red chili flakes
- ½ tsp. fennel seeds

- 3 tbsp. olive oil

Directions:

1. Switch on the air fryer, insert fryer basket, grease it with olive oil, then shut with its lid, set the fryer at 350°F and preheat for 5 minutes.
2. Open the fryer, add bacon strips in it, close with its lid and cook for 10 minutes until nicely golden and crispy, turning the bacon halfway through the frying.
3. Meanwhile, prepare the cabbage and for this, remove the outer leaves of the cabbage and then cut it into eight wedges, keeping the core intact.
4. Prepare the spice mix and for this, place onion powder in a bowl, add black pepper, garlic powder, salt, red chili, and fennel and stir until mixed.
5. Drizzle cabbage wedges with oil and then sprinkle with spice mix until well coated.
6. When the air fryer beeps, open its lid, transfer bacon strips to a cutting board and let it rest.
7. Add seasoned cabbage wedges into the fryer basket, close with its lid, then cook for 8 minutes at 400°F, flip the cabbage, spray with oil, and continue air frying for 6 minutes until nicely golden and cooked.
8. When done, transfer cabbage wedges to a plate.
9. Chop the bacon, sprinkle it over cabbage and serve.

BUFFALO CAULIFLOWER WINGS

Preparation Time: 5 minutes

Cooking Time: 20 minutes

Servings: 6

Nutritional values:

- Calories: 48 kcal
- Fat: 4 g
- Carbohydrates: 1 g
- Proteins: 1 g

Ingredients:

- 1 tbsp. almond flour
- 1 medium head of cauliflower
- 1 ½ tsp. salt
- 4 tbsp. hot sauce
- 1 tbsp. olive oil

Directions:

1. Switch on the air fryer, insert fryer basket, grease it with olive oil, then shut with its lid, set the fryer at 400°F and preheat for 5 minutes.
2. Meanwhile, cut cauliflower into bite-size florets and set aside.
3. Place flour in a large bowl, whisk in salt, oil, and hot sauce until combined, add cauliflower florets and toss until combined.
4. Open the fryer, add cauliflower florets in it in a single layer, close with its lid and cook for 15 minutes until nicely golden and crispy, shaking halfway through the frying.
5. When the air fryer beeps, open its lid, transfer cauliflower florets onto a serving plate and keep warm.
6. Cook the remaining cauliflower florets in the same manner and serve.

SWEET POTATO CAULIFLOWER PATTIES

Preparation Time: 20 minutes

Cooking Time: 25 minutes

Servings: 7

Nutritional values:

- Calories: 85 kcal
- Fat: 3 g
- Carbohydrates: 9 g
- Proteins: 2.7 g

Ingredients:

- 1 green onion, chopped
- 1 large sweet potato, peeled
- 1 tsp. minced garlic
- 1 cup cilantro leaves
- 2 cup cauliflower florets
- ¼ tsp. ground black pepper
- ¼ tsp. salt
- ¼ cup sunflower seeds

- ¼ tsp. cumin
- ¼ cup ground flaxseed
- ½ tsp. red chili powder
- 2 tbsp. ranch seasoning mix
- 2 tbsp. arrowroot starch

Directions:

1. Cut peeled sweet potato into small pieces, then place them in a food processor and pulse until pieces are broken up.
2. Then add onion, cauliflower florets, and garlic, pulse until combined, add remaining ingredients and pulse more until incorporated.
3. Tip the mixture in a bowl, shape the mixture into seven 1 ½ inch thick patties, each about ¼ cup, then place them on a baking sheet and freeze for 10 minutes.
4. Switch on the air fryer, insert fryer basket, grease it with olive oil, then shut with its lid, set the fryer at 400°F and preheat for 10 minutes.
5. Open the fryer, add patties in a single layer, close with its lid and cook for 20 minutes until nicely golden and cooked, flipping the patties halfway through the frying.
6. When the air fryer beeps, open its lid, transfer patties onto a serving plate, and keep them warm.
7. Cook the remaining patties in the same manner and serve.

OKRA

Preparation Time: 10 minutes

Cooking Time: 10 minutes

Servings: 4

Nutritional values:

- Calories: 250 kcal
- Fat: 9 g
- Carbohydrates: 38 g
- Proteins: 3 g

Ingredients:

- 1 cup almond flour
- 8 ounces fresh okra
- ½ tsp. sea salt
- 1 cup milk, reduced-fat
- 1 egg, pastured

Directions:

1. Crack the egg in a bowl, pour in the milk, and whisk until blended.
2. Cut the stem from each okra, then cut it into ½-inch pieces, add them into an egg and stir until well coated.
3. Mix flour and salt and add it into a large plastic bag.
4. Working on one okra piece at a time, drain the okra well by letting excess egg drip off, add it to the flour mixture, then seal the bag and shake well until okra is well coated.
5. Place the coated okra on a grease air fryer basket, coat the remaining okra pieces in the same manner, and place them into the basket.
6. Switch on the air fryer, insert fryer basket, spray okra with oil, then shut with its lid, set the fryer at 390°F and cook for 10 minutes until nicely golden and cooked, stirring okra halfway through the frying.
7. Serve straight away.

CREAMED SPINACH

Preparation Time: 10 minutes

Cooking Time: 20 minutes

Servings: 2

Nutritional values:

- Calories: 273 kcal
- Fat: 23 g
- Carbohydrates: 8 g
- Proteins: 8 g

Ingredients:

- ½ cup chopped white onion
- 10 ounces frozen spinach, thawed
- 1 tsp. salt
- 1 tsp. ground black pepper
- 2 tsp. minced garlic
- ½ tsp. ground nutmeg
- 4 ounces cream cheese, reduced-fat, diced
- ¼ cup shredded parmesan cheese, reduced-fat

Directions:

1. Switch on the air fryer, insert fryer basket, grease it with olive oil, then shut with its lid, set the fryer at 350°F and preheat for 5 minutes.
2. Meanwhile, take a 6-inches baking pan, grease it with oil and set it aside.
3. Place spinach in a bowl, add remaining ingredients except for parmesan cheese, stir until well mixed, and then, add the mixture into the prepared baking pan.
4. Open the fryer, add pan in it, close with its lid and cook for 10 minutes until cooked and cheese has melted, stirring halfway through.
5. Then sprinkle parmesan cheese on top of spinach and continue air fryer for 5 minutes at 400°F until top is nicely golden and cheese has melted.
6. Serve straight away.

CHEESY EGGPLANT

Preparation Time: 20 minutes

Cooking Time: 15 minutes

Servings: 4

Nutritional values:

- Calories: 193 kcal
- Fat: 5.5 g
- Carbohydrates: 27 g
- Proteins: 10 g

Ingredients:

- ½ cup and 3 tbsp. almond flour, divided
- 1.25-pound eggplant, ½-inch sliced
- 1 tbsp. chopped parsley
- 1 tsp. Italian seasoning
- 2 tsp. salt
- 1 cup marinara sauce
- 1 egg, pastured
- 1 tbsp. water

- 3 tbsp. grated parmesan cheese, reduced-fat
- ¼ cup grated mozzarella cheese, reduced-fat

Directions:

1. Slice the eggplant into ½-inch pieces, place them in a colander, sprinkle with 1 ½ tsp. salt on both sides, and let it rest for 15 minutes.
2. Meanwhile, place ½ cup flour in a bowl, add egg and water and whisk until blended.
3. Place remaining flour in a shallow dish, add remaining salt, Italian seasoning, and parmesan cheese, and stir until mixed.
4. Switch on the air fryer, insert fryer basket, grease it with olive oil, then shut with its lid, set the fryer at 360°F and preheat for 5 minutes.
5. Meanwhile, drain the eggplant pieces, pat them dry, and then dip each slice into the egg mixture and coat with flour mixture.
6. Open the fryer, add coated eggplant slices in it in a single layer, close with its lid and cook for 8 minutes until nicely golden and cooked, flipping the eggplant slices halfway through the frying.
7. Then top each eggplant slice with a tbsp. of marinara sauce and some of the mozzarella cheese and continue air frying for 1 to 2 minutes or until cheese has melted.

8. When the air fryer beeps, open its lid, transfer eggplants onto a serving plate, and keep them warm.
9. Cook remaining eggplant slices in the same manner and serve.

CAULIFLOWER RICE

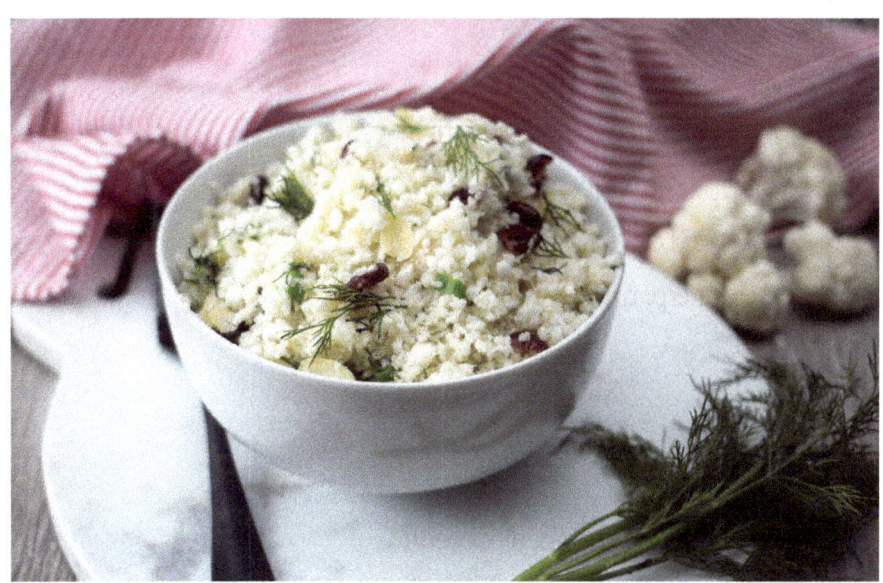

Preparation Time: 10 minutes

Cooking Time: 27 minutes

Servings: 3

Nutritional values:

- Calories: 258.1 kcal
- Fat: 13 g
- Carbohydrates: 20.8 g
- Proteins: 18.2 g

Ingredients:

For the Tofu:

- 1 cup diced carrot
- 6 ounces tofu, extra-firm, drained
- ½ cup diced white onion
- 2 tbsp. soy sauce
- 1 tsp. turmeric

For the Cauliflower:

- ½ cup chopped broccoli
- 3 cups cauliflower rice
- 1 tbsp. minced garlic
- ½ cup frozen peas
- 1 tbsp. minced ginger
- 2 tbsp. soy sauce
- 1 tbsp. apple cider vinegar
- 1 ½ tsp. toasted sesame oil

Directions:

1. Switch on the air fryer, insert fryer pan, grease it with olive oil, then shut with its lid, set the fryer at 370°F and preheat for 5 minutes.

2. Meanwhile, place tofu in a bowl, crumble it, then add remaining ingredients and stir until mixed.
3. Open the fryer, add tofu mixture in it, and spray with oil; close with its lid and cook for 10 minutes until nicely golden and crispy, stirring halfway through the frying.
4. Meanwhile, place all the ingredients for cauliflower in a bowl and toss until mixed.
5. When the air fryer beeps, open its lid, add cauliflower mixture, shake the pan gently to mix, and continue cooking for 12 minutes, shaking halfway through the frying.
6. Serve straight away.

DESSERT RECIPES

COCOA CAKE

Preparation Time: 10 minutes

Cooking Time: 22 minutes

Servings: 6

Nutritional values:

- Calories: 139 kcal
- Fat: 11 g
- Carbohydrates: 2 g
- Proteins: 4 g

Ingredients:

- Oz. butter
- 3 eggs
- 3 oz. sugar
- 1 tbsp. cocoa powder
- 3 oz. flour
- ½ tbsp. lemon juice

Directions:

1. Mix in 1 tbsp. butter with cocoa powder in a bowl and beat.
2. Mix in the rest of the butter with eggs, flour, sugar, and lemon juice in another bowl, blend properly and move half into a cake pan
3. Put half of the cocoa blend, spread, add the rest of the butter layer, and crest with remaining cocoa.
4. Put into the air fryer and cook at 360°F for 17 minutes.
5. Allow cooling before slicing.
6. Serve.

APPLE BREAD

Preparation Time: 10 minutes

Cooking Time: 46 minutes

Servings: 6

Nutritional values:

- Calories: 144 kcal
- Fat: 16 g
- Carbohydrates: 2 g
- Proteins: 9 g

Ingredients:

- 3 cups apples
- 1 cup sugar
- 1 tbsp. vanilla
- 2 eggs
- 1 tbsp. apple pie spice
- 2 cups white flour
- 1 tbsp. baking powder

- 1 stick butter
- 1 cup water

Directions:

1. Mix in egg with 1 butter stick, sugar, and apple pie spice, then turn using a mixer.
2. Put apples and turn properly.
3. Mix baking powder with flour in another bowl and turn.
4. Blend the 2 mixtures, turn, and move it to springform pan.
5. Get springform pan into the air fryer and cook at 320°F for 40 minutes
6. Slice.
7. Serve.

BANANA BREAD

Preparation Time: 10 minutes

Cooking Time: 42 minutes

Servings: 6

Nutritional values:

- Calories: 184 kcal
- Fat: 14 g
- Carbohydrates: 5 g
- Proteins: 4 g

Ingredients:

- ¾ cup sugar
- 1/3 cup butter
- 1 tbsp. vanilla extract
- 1 egg
- 2 bananas
- 1 tbsp. baking powder
- 1 and ½ cups flour
- ½ tbsp. baking soda

- 1/3 cup milk
- 1 and ½ tbsp. cream of tartar
- Cooking spray

Directions:

1. Mix in milk with cream of tartar, vanilla, egg, sugar, bananas, and butter in a bowl and turn whole.
2. Mix in flour with baking soda and baking powder.
3. Blend the 2 mixtures, turn properly, move into the oiled pan with cooking spray, put into the air fryer and cook at 320°F for 40 minutes.
4. Remove bread, allow to cool, slice.
5. Serve.

MINI LAVA CAKES

Preparation Time: 10 minutes

Cooking Time: 26 minutes

Servings: 3

Nutritional values:

- Calories: 165 kcal
- Fat: 18 g
- Carbohydrates: 2 g
- Proteins: 4 g

Ingredients:

- 1 egg
- 4 tbsp. sugar
- 2 tbsp. olive oil
- 4 tbsp. milk
- 4 tbsp. flour
- 1 tbsp. cocoa powder
- ½ tbsp. baking powder
- ½ tbsp. orange zest

Directions:

1. Mix in egg with sugar, flour, salt, oil, milk, orange zest, baking powder, and cocoa powder, turn properly. Move it to oiled ramekins.
2. Put ramekins in the air fryer and cook at 320°F for 20 minutes.
3. Serve warm.

CRISPY APPLES

Preparation Time: 10 minutes

Cooking Time: 10-15 minutes

Servings: 4

Nutritional values:

- Calories: 169
- Fat: 17 g
- Carbohydrates: 2 g
- Proteins: 2 g

Ingredients:

- 2 tbsp. cinnamon powder
- 5 apples
- ½ tbsp. nutmeg powder
- 1 tbsp. maple syrup
- ½ cup water
- 4 tbsp. butter
- ¼ cup flour

- ¾ cup oats
- ¼ cup brown sugar

Directions:

1. Get the apples in a pan, put in nutmeg, maple syrup, cinnamon, and water.
2. Mix in butter with flour, sugar, salt, and oat, turn, put a spoonful of the blend over apples, get into the air fryer and cook at 350°F for 10 minutes.
3. Serve while warm.